Lupus Recovery Diet

The Natural Lupus Recovery Solution

Table of Contents

Lupus – What exactly is it?

Lupus is a debilitating medical condition that some 1.5 million Americans suffer from, according to the Lupus Foundation of America. What makes it more frightening for people who develop the disease is that it has no cure, and you can only manage the condition in order to minimize organ damage and reduce the symptoms. Lupus is also tricky to diagnose, since its symptoms are similar to those of many other diseases, thus leading to its nickname "the great imitator". Because of this difficulty in identifying when a person has the disease, lupus often goes undiagnosed, which can be life-threatening. The Lupus Foundation estimates that there may be around 16,000 new cases every year.

What is Lupus?

Lupus is an autoimmune disease in which your body's immune system malfunctions and starts attacking healthy tissues rather than foreign substances such as viruses and germs. As a result of this condition, your body suffers damage in the joints and some of the internal organs. While there are three types of lupus, the most common form is Systemic lupus erythematosus (SLE). SLE can damage connective tissues in the joints and muscles as well as the membranes around the lungs, kidneys and heart. In addition, lupus may attack blood vessels which can cause sores or, in more serious cases, Reynaud's syndrome, in which the blood vessels to the feet and hands contract, resulting in blood being unable to reach the extremities. While attacks of Reynaud's last only a few minutes, they can be extremely painful and cause hands and feet to turn a bluish or white color.

Although anybody can develop lupus, women are most at risk, particularly when they are in their childbearing years. It is estimated that nine out of ten adults who suffer from lupus are women between the ages of fifteen to forty-five. Women with lupus are also at higher risk for developing the following conditions:

- Heart disease. Lupus patients are more prone to develop coronary artery disease, since they are more likely to have risk factors such as hypertension, type-2 diabetes and high cholesterol. In addition, since lupus sufferers are less physically active, they are at higher risk for heart disease.

- Osteoporosis. The medicines that are used to treat lupus may cause weaker bones and bone loss. In addition, since lupus patients are less likely to exercise, their bones may become more fragile.

- Kidney disease. Inflammation of the tissues around the kidney caused by lupus may affect the normal functioning of this organ. Kidney problems normally show up around five years after the onset of lupus symptoms. This is why people who suffer from lupus should have regular screenings of their kidney, in order to catch problems before they become more serious.

Certain races are also more likely to develop the disease, including Latinas, Asians, African-Americans and Native American women. For men, the ages when they are at the highest risk of developing lupus is before they reach the age of puberty and after fifty.

The Real Cause

While the exact cause of the disease is not known, it is believed that there are certain factors which may contribute to the development of lupus. These include:

- Family history. While having a close relative who has lupus may increase your risk for developing the condition, this is not necessarily the decisive factor. In fact, studies have shown that only 10% of lupus patients also have a sibling or parent with the disease.

- Negative environmental factors. Exposure to cigarette smoke, too much stress, spending too much time under the sun and certain viruses may cause the onset of lupus symptoms.

- Estrogen. It is believed that this hormone may cause some women in their prime childbearing years to develop lupus.

Early Signs of Lupus

There are a number of early signs that you may be suffering from lupus, which include:

- Fatigue. Ninety percent of lupus sufferers experience some degree of fatigue. While afternoon naps can help, too much sleeping during the day can cause insomnia at night. However, maintaining a daily routine can help keep your energy levels up so you can get by.

- Low-level fever. People with lupus can suffer from fevers between 98-degrees to 101-degrees F which has no apparent cause. If these fevers happen on a chronic basis, you should consult with a doctor.

- Thinning hair. People with lupus may notice their hair gradually falling out due to the inflammation of the skin on the scalp. In addition, hair may become brittle and break easily, which is referred to as 'lupus hair'.

- Skin rashes. One of the most visible signs that you may have lupus is butterfly-shaped rashes on the cheeks and the bridge of the nose. Some half of lupus sufferers develop these rashes, which can occur spontaneously or after exposure to sunlight. In some cases, the rashes may appear just before symptoms flare up.

- Nephritis. This is a kidney inflammation that makes it harder for the kidneys to perform their natural functions. People who have nephritis may experience hypertension and swelling of the feet and legs.

- Painful joints. Lupus may cause stiffness, pain and visible swelling in the joints, particularly during the morning.

Generally, people who have lupus do not experience symptoms all the time. There may be times when they feel fine, and then suddenly suffer from an outbreak. These outbreaks are known as "flares," and during these incidents, the symptoms become worse. These flares may be triggered by the following factors:

- Stress

- Lack of rest and working too hard

- Overexposure to the sun or to fluorescent lights

- Infections or injuries

- Certain medications

You should consult with your doctor if you experience several of these symptoms. If you have a family history of lupus, you should be more alert for the symptoms of the disease since you at a higher risk.

Lupus Diagnosis

Since there is no one test that can provide a clear diagnosis of lupus, doctors consider a number of factors including:

- Your medical history and those of close family members, including grandparents and aunts and uncles, in addition to your immediate family.

- The current symptoms that you are experiencing.

- Laboratory tests that can detect changes in the body which are consistent with a diagnosis of lupus. These tests those designed to detect antibodies which appear in a majority of lupus cases, such as ANAs, APLs, AntiRo (SSA) and AntiLA (SSB) and AntiSm as well as those looking for proteins that are involved in inflammation.

If one of more of these factors is positive, the doctor may come up with a diagnosis of lupus. If the doctor cannot come to a clear diagnosis, the patient may need to consult a rheumatologist. A rheumatologist is a specialist who treats patients with rheumatic diseases and helps them cope with their symptoms.

Conventional Treatment

There are a number of medications which are prescribed for people with lupus which treat some of the symptoms of the disease, which include:

- Non-steroidal anti-inflammatory drugs (NSAIDs) which treat muscle and joint pain in addition to inflammation. However, they may cause gastrointestinal problems such as stomach bleeding and pain.

- Corticosteroids which are intended to suppress the immune system in order to help reduce symptoms. These medications can cause serious side effects such as hypertension, osteoporosis, weight gain and cataracts, as well as increasing the risk of infection. Because of this risk, the dosage of the medication has to be closely regulated.

- Antimalarial medicines are intended to treat joint and skin problems related to lupus. While the risk of major side effects is minimal, these drugs may affect the eyes of people taking them. Thus, people taking antimalarial medications should have their eyes examined at least once a year to monitor for possible effects.

Lupus Flare Prevention

In addition to eating a more healthy diet, there are a number of recommended lifestyle changes that you should adopt which will also help keep your lupus under control. It should be noted that managing your lupus involves a holistic approach in which a good diet is combined with a healthier lifestyle.

- Stop smoking. Patients with SLE are already at a higher risk for developing heart disease, and smoking will only increase this risk further. In addition, smoking also prevents the most commonly-prescribed lupus medication from working.

- Learn to manage stress. Stress is acknowledged as one of the most common triggers of flares. There are a number of healthy ways that you can deal with stress. Becoming more physically active, such as taking long walks, for example, can help you de-stress after a long day. Learning how to meditate can help you relax and let go of stress. Seeking support from your loved ones can also be effective in reducing stress. If there is a support group for people with lupus in your area, you should consider joining since being with others who have the same affliction can help you cope with the disease better.

- Manage your energy. Since people who have lupus generally have less energy, they should learn how to manage it so that they can do what they need to without suffering from a flare. One of the things they should do is to not push themselves too hard and take a rest when they need to. Another is to not try to do too many things in a day. Finally, they should get enough sleep.

- Getting regular exercise. Exercise can help build up your strength and deal with lupus symptoms. You should develop a workout that includes these three types of workouts: range-of-motion, aerobic and strength training. These exercises can help you maintain normal joint movement, keep or increase muscle strength and improve overall fitness.

The Natural Treatment

People who have been diagnosed with lupus can manage their symptoms with a specialized diet. This diet will help you avoid flares by increasing your intake of foods that will not trigger symptoms of the disease. In addition, this diet will help you deal with the side effects caused by the medication prescribed to treat lupus symptoms. By adopting this specialized diet, along with the recommended lifestyle changes and regular treatment, you will be able to live a normal lifespan. In addition, the diet will also provide other wellness benefits such as helping you maintain a healthy weight and reducing the risk of developing other conditions such as heart disease and type-2 diabetes.

Here are some of the recommended guidelines to adopt when creating a healthy diet that will help you to control your lupus:

- Eat more foods with anti-inflammatory properties. Since lupus causes inflammation, adding more of these foods to your diet may help avoid flares and control your symptoms. Anti-inflammatory foods include: foods which are rich in antioxidants such as berries (strawberries and blueberries), beans (pinto and red kidney), apples, plums, prunes, artichokes and sweet cherries, as well as those which are high in Omega-3 fatty acids such as tuna and salmon, nuts, olive oil and ground flaxseed.

- Limit foods which are known to cause inflammation by increasing cholesterol levels. These include processed snack foods which are high in transfats, red meat, processed meat products such as salami and baloney, and dairy foods which are high in fat such as cheese, full-cream milk and ice cream. However, since the body still requires dairy to get its daily calcium requirements, you can shift to low-fat dairy alternatives, such as 1% skim milk, low-fat cheese and low-fat yoghurt. If you are lactose-intolerant, you can shift to soy milk or almond milk.

- One food that you should avoid is alfalfa sprouts. These vegetables are known to trigger symptom flares as well as causing a syndrome similar to lupus, which results in symptoms such as fatigue, kidney problems and muscle pain. While it is not known exactly why alfalfa triggers lupus symptoms, some researchers have theorized that the amino acid L-canavanine, which is present in alfalfa shoots and seeds, could turn on the immune system.

- In addition, avoid nightshade vegetables since they're known to cause inflammation. The nightshade vegetable family includes the following:

- Ashwagandha
- Bell peppers (a.k.a. sweet peppers)
- Bush tomato
- Cape gooseberry (also known as ground cherries—not to be confused with regular cherries)
- Cocona
- Eggplant
- Garden huckleberry (not to be confused with regular huckleberries)
- Goji berries (a.k.a. wolfberry)
- Hot peppers (such as chili peppers, jalapenos, habaneros, chili-based spices, red pepper, cayenne)

- Kutjera
- Naranjillas
- Paprika
- Pepinos
- Pimentos
- Potatoes (but not sweet potatoes)
- Tamarillos
- Tomatillos
- Tomatoes

Lupus Diet Recipe Ideas

Breakfast Ideas

Amazon Smoothie

Prep time: 5 minutes

INGREDIENTS

1 handful spinach

½ avocado

1 banana

1 large stalk celery

1 tsp cinnamon

1 cup water

INSTRUCTIONS

1. Slice avocado in half and remove the nut. Break the banana into small pieces and chop the celery into small pieces.
2. Combine all ingredients except for the spinach into a blender. Blend them until pureed, then add spinach and blend until pureed. Serve or chill and then serve.

Green Goodness Smoothie

Prep Time: 5 minutes

INGREDIENTS

2 cups spinach

2 whole kale leaves (1 cup chopped)

1 banana

1 green apple

1/2 cup green grapes

1 cup water (or fresh nut milk)

INSTRUCTIONS

1. Remove stems and ribs from kale. Core apple and dice. Peel banana.
2. Add water, banana and grapes to full sized blender. Process until solids are broken down.
3. Add greens and pulse on low for 30 seconds to break down. Then process on high for 1 minute, until smooth.
4. Pour into serving glasses and serve immediately.
5. Or chill in refrigerator for 20 minutes, blend for a few seconds to incorporate separated liquid, then pour into serving glasses and serve chilled.

Northern Typhoon

Prep time: 5 minutes

INGREDIENTS

1 handful Kale

1 banana

1 large cucumber

1 handful green beans

1 tsp cinnamon

1 cup water

INSTRUCTIONS

1. Break the banana into small pieces. De-stem the kale, skin and chop the cucumber and de-stem the green beans.
2. Combine all ingredients except for kale in a blender. Blend them until pureed, then add kale and blend until pureed. Serve or chill and then serve.

Pineapple Coconut Smoothie

Prep Time: 10 minutes*

INSTRUCTIONS

1 fresh coconut (or 1/2 cup flaked coconut)

1/2 cup pineapple chunks (fresh or frozen)

1 cup ice (crushed preferably)

Water

DIRECTIONS

1. *Soak flaked coconut in 1 1/2 cups water in refrigerator overnight, if using.
2. Add soaked coconut and soaking liquid to high-speed blender. Or remove flesh from fresh coconut and add to high-speed blender with 1 1/2 cups water. Process until well blended and fairly smooth, about 1 - 2 minutes.
3. Strain mixture through nut milk bag, cheesecloth or strainer back into blender.
4. Reserve pulp and set aside to dry and dehydrate, then use as coconut flour.
5. Cut pineapple flesh from peel, then chop. Add to blender with ice. Process until smooth, about 1 - 2 minutes.
6. Pour into serving glass and serve immediately.

Sweet Citrus Salad with Coconut Cream

Prep Time: 10 minutes

Servings: 1

INSTRUCTIONS

1 fresh coconut (or 1/2 cup flaked coconut)

1/4 - 1/3 cup dried pitted dates

1 blood orange

1 tangerine (or navel orange or clementine)

1/2 grapefruit (ruby red, pink or white)

1/2 lime

Water

INGREDIENTS

1. *Soak flaked coconut in 1 cup water overnight in refrigerator, if using. Soak dates in enough water to cover overnight in refrigerator. Drain.

2. Add soaked coconut and soaking liquid to high-speed blender. Or remove flesh from fresh coconut and add to high-speed blender with 3/4 cup water. Process until thick and fairly smooth, about 1 - 2 minutes.

3. Strain mixture through nut milk bag, cheesecloth or strainer back into blender or to food processor.

4. Reserve pulp and set aside to dry and dehydrate, then use as coconut flour.

5. Add soaked dates to processor and process until smooth. Set aside.

6. Peel all citrus and cut into segments. Add to serving dish. Top with sweet coconut cream.

7. Serve immediately. Or refrigerate 20 minutes and serve chilled.

Lunch and Dinner Ideas

Roasted Turkey Legs

Prep Time: 10 minutes*

Cook Time: 1 hour 20 minutes

Servings: 4

INGREDIENTS

2 large turkey legs

1/2 teaspoon garlic powder

1/2 teaspoon onion powder

1/2 teaspoon dried rosemary

1/2 teaspoon dried thyme

1/2 teaspoon sea salt

1 1/2 tablespoon coconut oil

Brine

4 cups water

1/4 cup sea salt

1/4 cup date butter

INSTRUCTIONS
1. *For *Brine*, add water, salt and date butter to wide, shallow container. Mix to combine. Add turkey legs and submerge completely in *Brine*. Marinate in refrigerator 12 - 24 hours.
2. Preheat oven to 350 degrees F. Place wire rack over sheet pan.

3. Remove turkey legs from brine. Rub salt, spices and oil over turkey legs, and under skin.

4. Place coated turkey legs on wire rack and bake about 35 - 40 minutes. Carefully turn turkey legs over and bake another 35 - 40 minutes, until skin is crisp and meat is cooked through.

5. Remove from oven and let rest about 2 minutes. Then serve hot.

Highland Beef Haggis

Prep Time: 10 minutes

Cook Time: 3 hours

Servings: 4

INGREDIENTS

8 oz (1/2 lb) ground beef (or bison, elk, etc.)

8 oz (1/2 lb) lamb shoulder

4 oz (1/4 lb) calves liver

2 onions (yellow or white)

1/2 head cauliflower (about 1 cup riced)

1 cup beef stock

2 garlic cloves

1/2 teaspoon ground nutmeg

1/4 teaspoon ground coriander

1/2 teaspoon sea salt

1/4 cup coconut oil

Water

INSTRUCTIONS

1. Preheat oven to 300 degrees F. Generously coat baking dish with coconut oil.

2. Add liver to small pan with enough water to cover over high heat. Bring to simmer and cook about 5 minutes. Drain and set aside to cool.

3. Roughly chop cauliflower. Peel and roughly chop onions and garlic. Add to food processor with lamb shoulder and par-cooked liver. Process until coarsely ground, about 2 minutes.

4. Add ground beef, stock, salt, and spices and pulse to combine. Transfer to prepared baking dish and cover tightly with aluminum foil.

5. Place covered dish in roasting pan. Add water to roasting pan 3/4 of the way up side of baking dish.

6. Bake for 3 hours. Remove from oven and carefully remove foil. Let rest about 10 minutes.

7. Remove baking dish from roasting pan. To plate, place serving dish over baking dish and carefully invert. Slice haggis into wedges and serve hot.

Bacon Wrapped Filet Mignon

Prep Time: 5 minutes

Cook Time: 20 minutes

Servings: 2

INGREDIENTS

2 (6 oz each) filet mignon steaks

2 thick slices nitrate-free bacon

sea salt, to taste

1 tablespoon coconut oil (optional)

Toothpicks

INSTRUCTIONS

1. Preheat oven to 350 degrees F. Heat medium oven-safe pan or skillet over medium heat.

2. Add bacon to hot pan. Cook and render out fat for about 5 minutes, until about halfway cooked. Remove bacon from pan and set aside, reserving bacon fat in pan. Add coconut oil to pan, if desired.

3. Wrap par-cooked bacon around steaks and secure with toothpick. Sprinkle steaks with salt to taste.

4. Add wrapped seasoned steaks to hot oiled pan and sear 2 minutes per side. Carefully flip half way through cooking.

5. Remove pan from stove and place in preheated oven. Cook about 8 - 10 minutes, until bacon is cooked through and steak is medium-rare.

6. Remove steaks from oven and transfer to cutting board. Set aside and let rest at least 2 minutes.

7. Transfer to serving dish and serve hot.

Herb Roasted Pork Tenderloin

Prep Time: 10 minutes*

Cook Time: 15 minutes

Servings: 4

INGREDIENTS

1 pork tenderloin

1 teaspoon dried rosemary

1 teaspoon dried thyme

1 teaspoon dried oregano

1 teaspoon dried basil

1 teaspoon dried marjoram (optional)

1 teaspoon sea salt

Apricot Sauce

1 cup dried apricots

2/3 cup water

1 teaspoon apple cider vinegar (or dry white wine)

INSTRUCTIONS

1. Preheat oven to 425 degrees F. Heat small pan over medium heat.
2. Rub tenderloin with salt and spices, then press into meat so it adheres. Place on sheet pan, or wire rack over sheet pan.
3. Roast for 10 - 15 minutes, until just cooked through and no pink remains. Remove pork from oven and let rest 10 minutes.

4. For *Apricot Sauce*, add dried apricots, water and vinegar to food processor or high-speed blender. Process until smooth, about 1 - 2 minutes.

5. Add *Apricot Sauce* to hot pan and reduce until slightly thickened. Stir well and do not let burn. Remove from heat.

6. Slice pork and transfer to serving dish. Top pork with *Apricot Sauce* and serve warm.

Classic Churrasco with Chimichurri

Prep Time: 10 minutes*

Cook Time: 5 minutes

Servings: 4

INGREDIENTS

24 oz (1 1/2 lb) beef tenderloin

Chimichurri

1 cup coconut oil

1/3 cup apple cider vinegar (or coconut aminos)

1/3 cup water

1 large bunch cilantro

1 large bunch parsley

1/2 cup fresh mint leaves

6 garlic cloves

1 teaspoon sea salt

INSTRUCTIONS

1. For *Chimichurri*, peel garlic and add to food processor or high-speed blender. Remove cilantro, parsley and mint leaves from stems. Add to processor and process to finely chop, about 1 minute. Add oil, water, salt and spices. Process until thick sauce forms, about 1 - 2 minutes.

2. Cut tenderloin lengthwise into 4 even slices, then flatten with tenderizing or kitchen mallet to 1/2 inch thickness. Place meat in between two parchment sheets to flatten, if preferred.

3. *Pour 1/4 of the *Chimichurri* into a baking dish just large enough to fit tenderloin. Place beef over *Chimichurri*, then top with second 1/4 of *Chimichurri*. Set aside to marinate about 1 hour. Transfer remaining *Chimichurri* to serving dish.

4. Heat grill or grated skillet over high heat.

Moist Roasted Turkey

Prep Time: 10 minutes*

Cook Time: 4 - 6 hours

Servings: 12

INGREDIENTS

20 lb (approx.) whole turkey

2 teaspoons sea salt

2 tablespoons coconut oil

Brine

1 - 2 gallons water

1 cup sea salt

1 cup date butter

INSTRUCTIONS

1. *For *Brine*, add 1/2 gallon of water, salt and date butter to large baking dish or roasting pan. Mix to combine. Remove any entrails from turkey and add to *Brine*, plus and enough water to submerge completely. Marinate in refrigerator 12 - 24 hours.

2. Preheat oven to 350 degrees F. Place roasting rack in clean roasting pan.

3. Drain turkey and rub salt and oil over and under skin, where possible.

4. Place seasoned turkey on roasting rack and bake about 15 - 18 minutes per lb, about 5 hours for 20 lb bird. Or until internal

temperature reaches 165 degrees F. Baste with rendered fat and juices throughout cooking for even browning.

5. Remove turkey from oven and let rest 20 - 30 minutes.
6. Carve and serve warm.

Quick Raw Avocado Slaw

Prep Time: 10 minutes*

Cook Time: 20 minutes

Servings: 4

INGREDIENTS

1/2 head cabbage (2 cups shredded)

1 avocado

1 carrot

Zest of 1 lemon

Juice of 1 lemon

1 tablespoon raw honey

2 tablespoons apple cider vinegar

1 teaspoon sea salt

INSTRUCTIONS

1. Cut avocado in half and remove pit. Scoop flesh into large mixing bowl and mash with fork.
2. Remove any tough outer leaves and core from cabbage. Shred cabbage and carrot. Add to bowl with vinegar, honey and salt. Zest *then* juice lemon, and add.
3. Toss to combine.
4. Serve immediately. Or and place in refrigerator for 20 minutes and serve chilled.

Snack Ideas

Smoked Salmon and Avocado Snack

Prep Time: 5* minutes

Servings: 2

INGREDIENTS

4 oz (1 or 1/2 package) cold-smoked salmon

1 avocado

1 stalk fresh dill

Pinch sea salt

1/2 lemon (optional)

INSTRUCTIONS

1. Slice avocado in half and remove pit. Cut into thick slices in peel then scoop out with large spoon.

2. Slice smoked salmon into long 1 inch strips. Wrap 1 salmon strips around each avocado slice. Arrange wrapped avocado on serving dish.

3. Mince fresh dill. Sprinkle dill and salt over avocado wraps and serve immediately.

4. Or squeeze juice of 1/2 lemon over avocado wraps, sprinkle on dill and salt, and refrigerate 20 minutes. Then serve chilled.

Olive Tapenade

Prep Time: 15 minutes

Servings: 2

INGREDIENTS

1 1/2 cups any combination pitted olives (Kalamata, Spanish, black, pimento, etc.)

2 tablespoons capers

2 anchovy fillets

1 garlic clove

2 fresh basil leaves

1/2 lemon

2 tablespoons coconut oil

INSTRUCTIONS

1. Peel garlic and add to food processor or high-speed blender. Process until finely ground.
2. Rinse and drain olives, capers and anchovy fillets. Add to processor with basil, oil and squeeze of 1/2 lemon. Process until finely chopped or coarsely ground, about 1 - 2 minutes.
3. Transfer to serving dish and serve immediately.

Tuna Tartare

Prep Time: 15* minutes

Servings: 4

INGREDIENTS

1 lb tuna steak (sushi grade)

1 small cucumber

1 ripe avocado

1 lime

1 garlic clove

2 tablespoons raw virgin coconut oil

Small bunch fresh cilantro

1 teaspoon sea salt

INSTRUCTIONS

1. Peel, seed and dice cucumber and avocado. Finely chop cilantro. Add to medium mixing bowl.
2. Peel garlic and add to food processor or bullet blender. Process until smooth paste forms. Add to bowl.
3. Dice tuna, discarding any tough white gristle. Add to bowl.
4. Squeeze on lime juice and add salt.
5. Gently toss with soft spatula or large spoon.
6. Serve immediately. Or refrigerate 20 minutes and serve chilled.

Baked Candied Yams

Prep Time: 10 minutes

Cook Time: 1 hour 30 minutes

Servings: 12

INGREDIENTS

4 large sweet potatoes (yams)

1/2 cup dried pitted dates

1/4 cup dried apricots

2 tablespoons coconut butter

1 tablespoon ground cinnamon

1/2 teaspoon ground ginger

Pinch sea salt

Topping

1/4 cup date butter

INSTRUCTIONS

1. Preheat oven to 350 degrees F.
2. Gently rinse sweet potatoes and place on sheet pan.
3. Bake about 1 hour, until tender.
4. Add dates, apricots and enough water to cover in small pot. Heat over medium heat. Let simmer until water evaporates. Remove from heat.
5. Remove yams from oven and let cool about 10 minutes.

6. For *Topping*, add date butter to small pan. Heat over medium heat and cook for about 4 - 5 minutes. Stir frequently and do not burn. Remove from heat and set aside.

7. Add softened dates and apricots to large mixing bowl. Mash with potato masher, hand mixer or whisk.

8. Cut yams open lengthwise and scoop flesh into mixing bowl. Add butter, salt and spices. Mash with potato masher, hand mixer or whisk until well combined.

9. Transfer yam mixture to serving dish and top with *Topping*. Serve warm.

Lean Mean Collard Greens

Prep Time: 15 minutes

Cook Time: 2 1/2 hours

Servings: 8

INGREDIENTS

2 heads (or 2 large bags) fresh collard greens

6 slices nitrate-free bacon (or 1 small ham hock)

8 cups chicken stock

Water

INSTRUCTIONS

1. Preheat oven to 350 degrees F. Heat large pot over medium-high heat.
2. Rinse collards well and roughly chop. Place in large colander or in clean sink to drain.
3. Add bacon or ham hock to hot pot and render down for about 5 minutes.
4. Add greens to pot in batches. If all greens to not fit, reserve. Add chicken stock.
5. Bring pot to a simmer then reduce to low heat. Add any remaining greens, plus enough water just to cover, if necessary. Stir gently.
6. Simmer until collards are tender, about 2 - 2 1/2 hours.
7. Drain greens well. Transfer to serving dish and serve warm.

5. Place beef on grill or skillet on the diagonal and cook for about 1 minute, then rotate meat to create crosshatch grill marks and cook

for another minute. Then flip and repeat. Cook for about 4 minutes total for medium rare.

6. Remove from grill, slice against the grain and transfer to serving dish. Serve immediately with *Chimichurri*.

Turkey Jerky Bacon

Prep Time: 10 minutes*

Dehydrating Time: 4 - 8 hours

Servings: 4

INGREDIENTS

4 oz organic turkey (dark meat)

2 tablespoons coconut aminos (or liquid aminos)

2 tablespoons tamari (or liquid aminos or coconut aminos)

1 tablespoon lemon juice (or raw apple cider vinegar)

1 tablespoons sea salt

1/2 teaspoon garlic powder

1/2 teaspoon onion powder

INSTRUCTIONS

1. Prepare two sheet parchment. Lay one on cutting board.
2. Cut turkey into 1/4 inch strips and lay in single layer on parchment. Pound with tenderizing side of kitchen mallet. Cover turkey with second parchment sheet, then pound with flat side of tenderizing mallet to 1/8 inch thickness.
3. *Place turkey strips in medium mixing bowl or shallow dish. Add coconut aminos, tamari, lemon juice, salt and spices. Mix well to coat. Cover and place in refrigerator for 8 hours, or overnight.
4. Remove turkey from refrigerator and lay in single layer on dehydrator trays. Place trays in dehydrator and set to 120 degrees F for 4 - 8 hours.

5. After 4 hours dehydrating time, remove trays from dehydrator and test turkey by bending. If it cracks, remove and serve immediately. Or store in airtight container.

6. If still flexible, place back in dehydrator and continue dehydrating up to 4 hours, or until desired texture is achieved.